WHITE

JOURNEY

The connection of science and medicine with philosophy and music

Volume I

The Tao of

Just About

Everything

by

Jeffrey Fisher

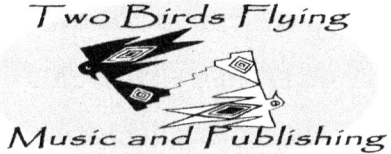

WHITE CLOUD JOURNEY

© JEFFREY FISHER 2010

ALL RIGHTS RESERVED

ISBN-13: 978-1461041016

ISBN-10: 1461041015

"A single step requires the journey of a thousand miles."

--Jeffrey Fisher, <u>Fractured Quotes</u>

To my teachers and students, and to the larger animal, plant and mineral family of which we are a part:

Remembering those who dug the well

from which we drink the water of truth;

those who planted the grapes

from which we press the wine

of progress;

and those who sow

the seeds of kindness

that replenish the Earth.

"Thus, the genetic code demonstrates convincingly and for all to see the difference between dualism and polarity, which has deceived us for centuries, since we have fallen into the trap of pure abstractions, fortified by logical conclusions that seem to prove the correctness lofty philosophical constructions and metaphysical speculations."

--Lama Govinda

"Tears of his Tears,

that turn the wheel of stars."

--the Zohar

CONTENTS

Part One. The Tao of Just About Everything—correlation of the three things, personal story

Preface: Music and Healing

Chapter 1. The Pattern of Life ... 12

Chapter 2. An Historical Note ... 15

Chapter 3. Synchronicity ... 17

Chapter 4. The Book of Changes ... 23

Chapter 5. Musical Scales and Hexagrams ... 36

Chapter 6. The Tao of Chaos ... 43

Chapter 7. DNA—Strands of Light ... 50

Part Two. Modes, Hexagrams and Amino Acids

Chapter 8. The Scales in Relation ...53

Part Three. What it All Means

Chapter 9. General principles…   77

Chapter 10. Snakes, evolution, prayer…

…83

Chapter 11. Holographic field   … 87

Chapter 12. The Triangle   … 90

Chapter 13. Activation   … 93

Chapter 14. Completion   … 97

PREFACE: Music and Healing

The time is the early 1990's. The place is a small village in Northern New Mexico. Though only fifty miles from the nearest fast food, stoplight or Wal-Mart—fifty rugged, forty-five-mile-per-hour, state-police-patrolled miles—the relative geographical isolation over the centuries has produced a kind of time warp for the inhabitants. They are very close-knit, very traditional. Descended from Spanish settlers from the Sixteenth Century, they have established a strong bond with the earth and this particular valley, which is between seven to nine thousand feet in elevation, surrounded by year-round snow-capped peaks. The winters are cold, but sunny; the summers green and relatively cool. My career as a jazz bassist is suspended for a few years until finding the musicians and clubs over the hill in Taos; I start composing albums for healing and massage background.

I also start teaching Tai Chi. My first students are cows and goats; soon, however, I have a class at the local drug and alcohol rehab center, and teaching at local communities—up to ninety miles away. As I begin to feel more at home in this "primitive" location, I realize that many of the ancient texts, including the Bible and the I-Ching, were written in this type of rural, simple environment, for these kinds of people, with their activities in mind.

As my involvement with Tai Chi grows, through teaching, practice and frequent trips to the big cities for advanced classes and workshops, I begin to realize the incredible potential of the art, especially for healing, and to feel the connection between music and the healing energy activated through Tai Chi practice. Over the next several years, they would merge even more. I train in Reiki/Reflexology/Acupressure, later in Auricular Medicine, and create the record label Healing Music of the Southwest and Two Birds Flying Tai Chi, Music and Publishing.

At this time, in the 1990's, there is an explosion of New Age music; musicians release many albums claiming to be "healing." Perhaps it is the rash of such albums that prompts the publication of an article in a New Age journal concerning healing and music. The writer of the article, in trying to be objective or "scientific," concludes that there is no real proof of the healing effects of music…any music. This, despite the fact that we have long been aware of the strong affect that certain types of music have on plants, animals and humans.

Science vs. Reality

This book is not intended to be a scientific treatise. It presents no scientific criteria necessary to "prove" anything (besides proving the fact that the author is not a scientist). I will present, however, information that will indicate a connection between music and healing. More precisely, I will show that a mathematical correlation exists between your DNA and the music you listen to every day.

The Tao and the Language of Consciousness

The discovery of this correlation is the story of the Tai Chi experience. It is also a personal story. It involves a coming together of people and ideas that have traveled across three continents and at least thirty centuries.

The word Tao is often translated as "the way" or "the path" or simply "truth." We have no word in English for the word Tao. However, a hidden word may shed some light, or at least cast some interesting shadows. That word is "groove," from which we get "groovy" (*adj., slang, "cool," "beatific," "far out"*). The groove is what we fall into when we are on the right path. It is not necessarily perfection. To paraphrase the Bhagavad-Gita, it is better to live one's own life imperfectly than to live someone else's perfectly. Why should we doubt that our lives are not ultimately going to lead us to truth, no matter how strange or convoluted the journey?

PART ONE:

THE TAO OF JUST ABOUT EVERYTHING

Chapter 1.

The Pattern of Life

Patterns and Puzzles

Did you ever wonder if your life was part of some large overall pattern or design? Or think that the most chance meeting of people or events was not accidental?

Patterns make up a large part of who, how and what we are. Our minds seem to have a natural proclivity to seek patterns out of chaos. The simple principles of Unity and Variety form the basis of our creative and communication process.

The question of why and how this occurs may not seem especially relevant, as it is buried in the infinite mirrored process we call the Oneness of all Things. Yet, our present field of inquiry treads dangerously close to the border of the mystery in which those particular riddles are hidden.

Perhaps it is what people call the Tao; perhaps it is what modern scientists call the Implicate Order—the ineffable, indefinable and unreachable essence that defies reason. Nowadays, we have the Tao of many things—physics, medicine, Pooh, mortgage refinancing. Taos, like healing modalities, are rampantly multiplying and patented every few hours. However, the Tao of Just About Everything concerns only three things, at least two of which have been around since ancient times:

                1. The genetic code

2. Music   3. The I-Ching

The language of consciousness

What does an ancient Chinese book of philosophy have to do with the equally old mathematical theories describing music and the relatively recent discoveries of what is contained within the nucleus of a living cell?

These three seemingly unrelated areas of thought not only have a relationship to each other; they have a complete and absolute correlation. The discovery of this correlation—the author's personal adventure—is a small story strewn with uncommon synchronicities amidst a huge ocean of more intriguing explorations, including the bizarre tragedy and high drama associated with the origin of the I-Ching.

Chapter 2.
An Historical Note

Before the Beginning

Our story begins in China, or that part of the world later known as China. Who really knows where this story begins, or when? Legend has it that Fu Hsi, a semi-mythological figure from the era of hunting and fishing and the inventor of cooking and language, is sitting on the bank of a river pondering the patterns on the back of a tortoise. He thus brings forth the eight Trigrams that became the basis for the I-Ching, the Book of Changes.

The Shang Emperor Chou Hsin

By the time of the Shang Emperors, around 1150 BC, the eight Trigrams have already been discovered, explained and codified. King Wen, who is not yet a king (the title was given to him posthumously), is head of a western state that is under the oppressive rule of the Shang Emperor, who is, even for his day, a brutal tyrant. (One winter day, upon seeing peasants up to their knees in the freezing rice paddies, he wonders how they can stand the cold. He is said to have ordered their legs cut off to find out if they were constructed differently.)

King Wen Writes I-Ching After Dinner

At the Emperor's court, after an unusually cruel and heartless punishment is meted out, King Wen was heard to sigh audibly. This gesture of compassion earned him a jail cell where this Emperor Chou Hsin forced him to eat soup made from his oldest son. It was in this period of incarceration that King Wen composed the judgments to the Hexagrams. His other son, the Duke of Chou, later added more to the I-Ching and overthrew Chou Hsin. He started his own dynasty, the Chou Empire, which lasted until 249 BC (close to one thousand years!)

Chapter 3.
Synchronicity

The Town Where Nothing Ever Happened

In 1985, I cease being a hippie jazz musician in Berkeley and move to Los Angeles to study composing and film scoring. At the Grove School of Music in Studio City, we are given the assignment to write the opening theme for a television show—any show. Since I still do not watch television, I make up my own show.

Television Series: "The Town Where Nothing Ever Happens"—OPENING SEGMENT:

As the sound of the first dramatic chord of the theme, the camera pans on the horizon: a desert sunrise—growing contrast of light and dark. As the camera pans 180 degrees and light builds, we start to make out a small town on the edge of the desert, the highway running through it. Zooming through the town, we see just how small it is. There are no people, only a couple of parked cars on the street. A dog walks across the street and urinates on the building where the majority of the action will take place: A Sears Catalogue Store. As the segments progress, we see strange synchronicities occurring to the protagonists, who are marginally involved with an elderly person of Asian descent who possesses unusual psychic abilities.

Three years later, due to a series of fateful quirks, I find myself living in that town.

This is not strange in itself, since I grew up there. It is unusual, though, that the legendary and charismatic Dr. Marshall Ho'o has moved to the area and is teaching at a local senior center. I have had some previous training in Tai Chi Chuan in Berkeley, and find Dr. Ho'o's classes physically unchallenging and to be bordering on dull. I have no idea that the 82 year-old Dr. Ho'o was in the Black Belt Hall of Fame, that created the National Tai Chi Chuan Association and sponsored some of the first Chinese teachers to teach Americans, and that the governor of California designated his birthday Marshall Ho'o Day for his work in getting Acupuncture certified in the state.

Irony Waves

All of this I learn much later. At first, I am not actually impressed with him. Who expects to find greatness in their hometown? Many times, I fall asleep in his lectures, fascinating as they are. At this time, I am not especially interested in "finding a guru," though in previous years that search has been in the back of my mind. It is one of life's ironies that often when we do get what we wish for that we have either stopped wishing for it or are too busy to notice. Often, I complain to friends that Dr. Ho'o would just sit and read instead of preparing lessons for his acupuncture class. It is years later, when studying on my own and more in depth that I realize the books from which he was reading are so rare that I could never hope to find them.

Tai Chi Chuan and Dr. Ho'o

At the time, I have very little idea how important this man will be in my own life, let alone how many hundreds—and through his students, thousands—of followers he has. It is important to note that it is not his personality or guruness that makes Dr. Ho'o important to so many people. Two things make him exceptional. One is the fact that he is Chinese-American—Chinese enough for those who thought Americans unworthy or unable to understand Tai Chi to teach him the real thing, and American enough to communicate with the young people of the 1960's through the 1980's. The second fact is that his teaching, his love and understanding of Tai Chi comes from the heart as well as the mind and body. His teaching seemed to pour through his entire being.

My experience in learning Tai chi from Dr. Ho'o turns out to be more than just an interesting class to fill up my time or "a hobby." I find an opening to a new and complete field of knowledge—something for which I have been searching since my first glance at a college catalogue. (I started out as a theatre major at a small private college noted for academic excellence but which also had a heavily endowed theatre department. Theatre was as close as I could come at the time to a field of training and knowledge that trained the whole person). As I become closer to Dr. Ho'o and his partner Strawberry Gatts—now both deceased—I find my interest and commitment to Tai Chi deepening enormously. Soon, it would get <u>very</u> interesting, as I realize the potential for a personal art form developed over thousands of years.

Tai Chi Chuan and the I-Ching

In Tai Chi class one day, Dr. Ho'o mentions the Three Pillars of Tai chi Chuan: the Acupuncture system, the philosophies of Buddhism, Taoism and Confucianism and the I-Ching. That the I-Ching was one of the foundations of Tai Chi Chuan I found very interesting. Many of my contemporaries carried an I-Ching around for years, consulting it about everything from moving to jobs and relationships. Intriguing that it could form the basis for martial arts and exercise!

My own copy of the Book of Changes, purchased at Samuel Weiser's in New York when I was nineteen, has traveled with me across the country and state-to-state many times. But where is it? I have just moved. Have I unpacked it? With the thought of dozens of unpacked boxes waiting for me in the garage, I walk across the street to the bookstore that has opened just the week before, not really expecting to find the I-Ching among the Microwave Cookbooks and dog-eared Reader's Digest Condensed Books. This is, after all, still the "town where nothing (much) ever happens."

However, to my surprise, there it is! Opening the cover for a price, I see that indeed, it is my own copy had mistakenly fallen into an estate sale at my parent's house the previous year.

So, reunited with the I-Ching, I make an interesting discovery; but it will take another nine years for the importance of the discovery to unfold.

Chapter 4. The Book of Changes

Yin and Yang and Taoism

Ages ago, people noticed that everything has a front and a back, was either hot or cold, male or female, etc. and sensed that there were two forces at work in the universe. These, they called Yin and Yang, the two opposite polarities in the universe from which springs everything else.

This is the basis of the philosophy of Taoism. The Tao—(pronounced *dow*)—is defined as that which cannot be defined, but loosely discussed as "the way" or " the truth." So, the abstract and infinite is based on something (Yin and Yang) that is concrete and definite.

Yin and Yang of the I-Ching and Computers

In the I-Ching, Yang, symbolizing the positive force in the universe, is represented by a solid line (—). The negative force is represented by a broken line (--). Yin and Yang, however, are not true opposites, but two aspects of the same energy.

Modern computers based on a system much like this—called the binary code—owe their existence to the German mathematician Leibnitz. His binary mathematics uses only two numbers, 0 and 1. Subsequent to the invention of this system, Leibnitz read the I-Ching and realized that his work had been accomplished hundreds of years previously.

Just as the binary system uses but two numbers to describe anything from the simplest to the most complex of mathematical situations, a computer uses tiny little switches that are either ON or OFF to represent the complexity of words or images, and the I-Ching uses the solid (—) and broken (--) lines to describe the complexity of the universe. This is expressed in layers, stacking lines one on top of the other, in groups of three, producing eight different possibilities:

THE TAO OF JUST ABOUT EVERYTHING

The Eight Trigrams

CH'IEN / THE CREATIVE   K'UN / THE RECEPTIVE   CHEN / AROUSING   K'AN / ABYSMAL

KEN / KEEPING STILL   SUN / GENTLE   LI / FIRE, CLINGING   TUI / JOYOUS

These Trigrams represent forces or processes in nature; they are symbols of transitional states of movement, of change. Stacked with one another, they create an even greater multiplicity of meanings—the 64 Hexagrams.

THE 64 HEXA-GRAMS

THE TAO OF JUST ABOUT EVERYTHING

1. The Creative

2. The Receptive

3. Difficulty at Beginning

4. Youthful Folly

5. Waiting/Nourishment

6. Conflict

7. The Army

8. Holding Together/Union

9. Taming Power of the Small

THE TAO OF JUST ABOUT EVERYTHING

10. Treading/Conduct   11. Peace   12. Standstill/Stagnation

13. Fellowship with Men   14. Possession in Great Measure   15. Modesty

16. Enthusiasm   17. Following   18. Decay

THE TAO OF JUST ABOUT EVERYTHING

19. Approach

20. Contemplation/View

21. Biting Through

22. Grace

23. Splitting Apart

24. Return/Turning Point

25. Innoncence/Unexpected

26. Taming Power of the Great

27. Corners of the Mouth/ Providing Nourishment

THE TAO OF JUST ABOUT EVERYTHING

28. Preponderance of the Great   29. The Abysmal/Water   30. Clinging/Fire

31. Influence/Wooing   32. Duration   33. Retreat

34. Power of the Great   35. Progress   36. Darkening of the Light

THE TAO OF JUST ABOUT EVERYTHING

37. The Family

38. Oppposition

39. Obstruction

40. Deliverance

41. Decrease

42. Increase

43. Breakthrough/
Resoluteness

44. Coming to Meet

45. Gathering Together

THE TAO OF JUST ABOUT EVERYTHING

46. Pushing Upward

47. Oppression/Exhaustion

48. The Well

49. Revolution/Moulting

50. The Cauldron

51. Arousing/Thunder

52. Keeping Still/Mountain

53. Development/
Gradual Progress

54. The Marrying Maiden

THE TAO OF JUST ABOUT EVERYTHING

55. Abundance/Fullness   56. The Wanderer   57. Gentle/Penetrating/Wind

58. Joyous/Lake   59. Dispersion/Dissolution   60. Limitation

61. Inner Truth   62. Preponderance of the Small   63. After Completion   64. Before Completion

The Question

The sixty-four Hexagrams are patterns formed with six solid and/or broken lines. Though representative of the possibilities and permutations of human life and living, that particular afternoon I am only concerned with the pattern itself. The six solid or broken lines seem an interesting way of notating musical scales. How can a seven-note scale be represented by a 6-line hexagram?

Chapter V. Musical Scales and Hexagrams

Musical Scales

To understand music, it is only necessary to look at a piano keyboard. We see that it has black keys and white keys in a certain repeating order of five black and seven white. The seven white notes are named A, B, C, D, E, F and G; then it starts again.

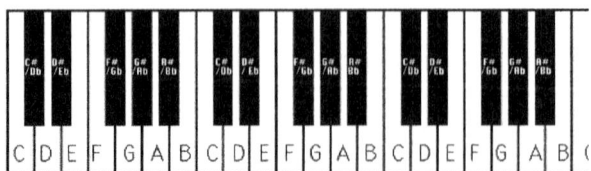

Playing solely the white keys starting on C, one produces the very familiar sound of the major scale:

C D E F G A B C

Or :

Do Re Mi Fa So La Ti Do

This seemingly simple arrangement of notes is not only imbedded in our collective and individual consciousness, it also represents a keystone of an ancient system for unlocking the mystery of all that is. For now, we will simply observe the pattern of white and black notes.

The Black Notes

We note that there are black notes in between all the white notes except E and F and between B and C. This makes the <u>interval</u> between these notes smaller than the notes that have a black key in between.

Whole Steps and Half Steps

The larger interval—two white keys with a black key in between (or two black keys with a white key in between)—is a *whole step.* The smaller interval—between any white key and an adjacent black key (or between E and F or B and C)—is a *half step*.

The Pattern of a Major Scale (the white notes)

The major scale then is:

```
     Whole        Whole       half
C     ^      D     ^      E  ^  F
```

Whole

```
       Whole     Whole      half
   ^  G    ^   A    ^     B  ^  C
```

Dividing the Scale

Leaving aside for a moment the question of why we might want to do this, we can divide the scale into two equal parts:

CDEF and GABC.

The Greek philosopher Pythagoras, known for his astute mathematical observations, called these scale fragments *tetra chords*. (*tetra* = four).

The intervals between the notes in these two particular tetra chords are:

Whole   Whole   Half   and
Whole   Whole   Half:

C ^ D   ^ E ^ F   and

G ^ A   B ^ C

That is, *six* intervals.

Using the I-Ching solid and broken lines with which we are already familiar, **a half step can be indicated by a yin or broken line, the whole step by a Yang or sold** line, and the major scale would look like this:

```
━━━  ━━
━━━━━
━━━━━
━━━  ━━
━━━━━
━━━━━
```

58. Joyous/Lake

Starting on a different note within the same scale produces a different-sounding scale, and a different Hexagram. The same C major scale starting from A would look like this:

    Whole   *Half*   *Whole*

A   ^ *B* ^ *C* ^ *D*

    Half   *Whole*   *Whole*

$E \quad \wedge \quad F \quad \wedge \quad G \quad \wedge \quad A$

Again, the larger interval, the whole step, would correspond to a solid line, the smaller interval, the half step, would correspond to a broken line. The scale starting on A could be represented by this Hexagram:

```
━━━━━━
━━━━━━
━━  ━━
━━━━━━
━━  ━━
━━━━━━
```

37. The Family

These seven white notes, in the same order, can be spelled out seven different ways:

CDEFGABC

DEFGABCD

EFGABCDE

FGABCDEF

GABCDEFG

ABCDEFGA

BCDEFGAB

These are the seven modal variations of the major scale; they form the basis of much of the world's music.

On a single page of manuscript paper, I write out these seven modal variations of the major scale and its corresponding Hexagrams. Though I find it interesting and may even show it to a couple people, it goes in the drawer for many years. After all, who cares that you can write a musical scale using a series of solid and broken lines? People have enough trouble reading the system of notation that has come down to us from who knows where, yet alone playing those scales. It is years later, through a chance conversation with another of Marshall Ho'o's students about Chaos Theory, that the wheel comes around, and the Tao of just about everything is born.

Chapter 6. "Tao of Chaos"

Chaos Theory and the I-Ching

Chaos theory developed through the study of weather patterns. As a system becomes increasingly complex, it approaches a state of chaos.

An example would be a glass of water. If the glass is left on the table, the molecules are in a predictable order. As soon as the glass is picked up, the molecules start to move. If the glass is swirled gently in a circle, the water is still unspilled and predictable within certain limits. If the swirling gets too vigorous, the water spills, having reached a point of chaos.

Human events, relationships and behaviors can be simple, or they can be as complex and unpredictable as the weather. This progress from simplicity to complexity is mirrored in the Hexagrams of the I-Ching. The first line can be one of two possibilities, yin or yang, broken or solid. It could also be a *changing line*, making it one of four possibilities; that is, if three coins are tossed to determine each line, one of four possibilities will occur:

It will either be two heads and a tail (Yang line); two tails and a head (Yin line); all heads (Yang *changing* line); or all tails (Yin *changing* line). The first line can have only four possibilities. However, in combination with the first line, the number of possibilities for the second line is 16; for the third line 256; fourth line 65536, fifth 4,249,967,296; the sixth the square of that, 18,253,470,545,389,551,616.

In digital graphic technology, there is a point at which the number of dots per square inch gives us an acceptable image of reality; the more dots, the more "real" it looks. In digital sound recording technology, a certain sampling rate will give us an approximation of the sound of a violin, for example, that we will be able to distinguish from the sound of a toy harmonica; the higher the sampling rate, the more "real." We might also say that this number 18,253,470,545,389,551,616 (four to the sixth power), which is the total number of I-Ching possibilities, approximates reality in a certain way. It also approaches the chaos inherent in reality. However, since it is merely an approach or approximation and *not* random, we might also say that the I-

Ching also gives us an order beneath, or enfolded into the randomness.

This implicate order has been discovered by mathematicians within random series of numbers, such as the Mandelbrot Set. What appears to be a mathematically random series of numbers, when plotted on a pixelled screen, forms an image. This image, when magnified, shows a repetition of a pattern seen in the first image, but on a smaller scale. These repetitions of the same pattern through different orders of magnitude seem to persist infinitely.

This order is expressed also by the fractal geometry present on all levels in our natural world; for instance, the shape and number of leaves on a tree; the digits in a hand or paw; the shape of a coastline or a mountain range. In fact, just about everything.

The DNA to I-Ching Connection

It turns out that the number of Hexagrams in the I-Ching, is a significant number. In *The Tao of Chaos,* Ms. Walter has discovered a connection between the sixty-four I-Ching Hexagrams with the sixty-four amino acid permutations in the DNA. This is something people have been toying with for a few years now—after all, sixty-four permutations of _anything_ (Crayolas aside) is not so common.

The difference is that Ms. Walter discovered an absolute correlation of the meanings of the Hexagrams to the function of the amino acid in the body. For instance, the I-Ching Hexagram # 58 Shared Joy corresponds to the molecule Serine. Serine regulates the connection between the brain and nervous system. We will see in Part Two of this book how close this is to the meaning of "Shared Joy" as expressed in the I-Ching.

Reading more of the I-Ching commentaries and comparing them to the various Amino Acids, the truth of Dr. Walter's premise becomes clear. In other words, an ancient book of philosophy contains encrypted information that relates directly to what we have very recently learned about the very specific functioning of DNA in our bodies. This would seem to validate not only the I-Ching, but the work done on identifying the amino acids and their function.

The Music/I-Ching/DNA Connection

Very shortly after coming into contact with The Tao of Chaos, out of curiosity I look up my old notes on the scales and Hexagrams.

Interestingly enough, I find Hexagram # 58, Shared Joy corresponded in my system to the major scale.

▬▬ ▬▬
▬▬▬▬▬
▬▬▬▬▬
▬▬ ▬▬
▬▬▬▬▬
▬▬▬▬▬

58. Joyous/Lake

:

= **C D E F G A B C**

It would not be difficult to argue that the major scale, even if Beethoven's "Ode to Joy" had never been written, is a happy sound. Reading the commentaries on this Hexagram in the I-Ching is enlightening to the musician, as it clearly could be talking about the construction and nature of this scale. In Chapter 8 on the Modes and Hexagrams, the reader will find a more complete discussion of this and other scales in relation to the meaning of the Hexagrams. In some cases the connection is glaring; in other cases, one has to take more steps (or leaps) to find the connection.

Accidental purpose

On one hand, this book is accidental, as I would probably never thought to have looked for that specific correlation between the emotional qualities of a particular scale and the meaning of the Hexagrams. On the other hand, it maybe more astounding because I <u>was not</u> looking for them. However, there is nothing accidental about the connection among these seemingly disparate areas of knowledge; and it leads us to wonder if there are not many more connections that we are missing, some of which may solves some interesting problems or lead to important breakthroughs in thought and science and technology.

A triangle is formed, a connection between or among three dramatically different areas of knowledge. On one corner is the genetic code, on the other is the I-Ching and on the third angle is music—but why is it important?

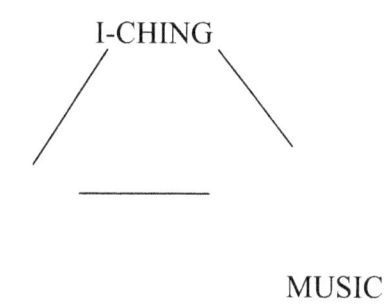

```
           I-CHING
          /       \
         /         \
        /           \
       /   _____     \

    DNA              MUSIC
```

Apparently, three areas of study—the I-Ching, the genetic code and music—share a common language. In the middle of the triangle lies perhaps a commonality that is beyond language. It is the language of consciousness itself, the Tao of just about everything.

Chapter 7. DNA – Strands of Light

The Past Within the Future

The DNA is the repository of genetic information—the past, present and future of humanity and the individual. Each cell contains the information to create not only a whole individual, but also information of the entire human species. The DNA has to create a human being before it makes a specific individual. In reality, since DNA is contained in every living thing, the information *life itself* is in each cell.

Yet the DNA does even more than that: by communicating to its sister strands the RNA, it forms the chemicals that have everything to do with the day to day, moment to moment processes of life. That is what an amino acid is. Every function of the body, every thought and feeling is some how connected to this basic matrix of sixty-four possibilities. The last chapter explained how those sixty-four possibilities relate to the larger matrix:

18,253,470,545,389,551,616.

The Scale of Scales

Coincidentally, we have also arrived at a number of harmonically stable musical scales of seven notes. Do we really need all those scales? Like the "Old Woman in the Shoe," we would have so many scales we would be chasing them around all the time and not being extremely productive (though it might be good to not be afraid one would ever run out). There is good reason to believe that we will continue to use the same old fragments of tone combinations that have bounced off each other for eons, undoubtedly for the same reason that our amino acids are limited and that we supposedly only use a fraction of our brains.

More to the point is what I would call activation and mastery. Activation is the subject of Volume Two of this book; it is the process of unenfoldment of inherent potential. Mastery, rather than being comprehensive and expansive to the nth degree, is simply mastering the basics and applying them with utmost clarity. (Think of John Coltrane and his "sheets of sound"—you can still hear the basic chord structure, you can still hear the blues; think of Beethoven's symphonies where he has pared down to the point that there is no difference between form and structure.)

Though the musician may glean from these pages some new understanding and materials with which to work, he or she already knows that music has an emotional and healing impact. The fact of the connection to non-musical areas may or may not be of interest. There also may exist the potential for a musical "system." I will leave that as well for others to create, as I believe all systems to be false—even if true…especially if true.

Along the musical path, an interesting question can be more useful than someone else's explanation or answer. I seek to widen the field of possibilities, not to reveal any great secret.

We are all musicians

Consciously or consciously, we are all musicians. We manipulate our environment—which consists of vibrations—to be more pleasing to all. We start with the more subtle vibrations of emotion and idea and progress by any means possible through stages of physical manifestation. We have seen in these pages how much of the patterns of our lives are connected and related to each other. It is the recognition of these patterns that can determine whether something is pleasing to the eye, ear or mind, or has some emotional impact. In search of freshness, composers have attempted to fight these constraints and created music based solely on chance. To think that it could be the brain alone that creates music!

PART TWO.

Modes, Hexagrams and Amino Acids

Chapter 8. Musical scales and I-Ching hexagrams

Using the note C as a starting point, though any of the twelve notes could be used, we will examine the Hexagrams and their relationship to specific scales and amino acids. The information on the amino acids and their correspondence to the Hexagrams is all from <u>The Tao of Chaos</u> by Katya Walter; I have discussed only those amino acids of which she makes specific mention. However, you will find included many scales for which the amino acid correlation is missing; the musician and non-musician alike may find these interesting. Quotes from the I-Ching are from the Wilhelm/Baynes Edition.

A complete discussion of the amino acid connection is beyond the scope of this book. Relating the scales to a particular Hexagram sometimes consists in speculative leaps and subjective discernments, but I believe there is enough truth here to warrant the exercise.

In this context, please note there are three different kinds of scales. First, there are THE MODES, the standard permutations of the major diatonic scale; secondly, ALTERED SCALES, which are in common use in classical European and classic jazz music; thirdly, ASYMMETRICAL SCALES, which do not come back around to the starting note in the next octave, for instance:

CDEF GABC#

These scales are more spirals than circles; they are useful nonetheless. The term symmetrical refers not to a scale that is not asymmetrical, but to a scale whose tetra chords both have the same structure; for example: CDEF# / GABC#.

Is there a point to examining these scales? It is that we may wish to progress in our music beyond the merely pretty or pleasing into the realm of real meaning. It is a fleeting vision. We are not necessarily looking for a concrete correlation or anything so concrete as the raga system, where a particular scale represents a certain time of day, or feeling--nothing so simplistic as an absolute correlation, such as saying that a major scale must always be happy.

When I refer to meaning, what I mean is *reality*—what is beyond words. I hope by means of this exercise to learn more of the structure of music; how the notes affect each other. The lesson of Beethoven: how he combined form with meaning (not literal meaning, but emotional meaning). Everything we can think or feel can be expressed musically. As we combine our thoughts and feelings with a musical construction, then we have achieved some form of musical truth. These musical constructions must be recognized only intuitively; if we look them up in a list somewhere, we will never be sure of the result. However, the mind does start to learn patterns and meanings; the ear forms associations. We can only listen, and understand.

Hexagram 1: The Creative

C D E F# G A B C#

The power of pure spirit; the power of time and the power of persisting in time.

All of the scales have to be experienced to be understood. This Hexagram carries the implication of *self-development.* "...there is also created the idea of duration both in and beyond time, a movement that never stops nor slackens, just as one day follows another in an unending course.........With this image as a model, the sage learns how best to develop himself so that his influence may endure." To me, this suggests that at least in this symmetrical scale, we must use it to explore all twelve keys. We will extend from the C# and start the same pattern on D; then, on E, F#, G#, and A#. Since the scale consists of two identical tetra chords a fifth apart composed solely of whole steps, in starting the scale six times, we have completed the circle of 5ths. Most musicians are aware of the power of the circle of 5ths. Not only the tuning of stringed instruments (the violin and guitar families), but the sequence of 90% of chord sequences follow this pattern in some way. Besides learning the names of the notes and to play a major scale, the circle of 5ths is the most powerful tool the musician has.

Please also note that the concept of time discussed by the I-Ching on Hexagram 1 is the same concept instilled in musicians—of metrical time as an independent force, each beat given the exact same duration. All stretching is within that implied metrical framework. This allows musicians to play together cohesively.

Hexagram 2: The Receptive

C Db Eb Fbb   G Ab Bbb Cbb

Phenoalynine

Being composed of broken lines only, this Hexagram represents the primal power of Yin. Its attribute is devotion. In the Tai Chi game of push-hands, the principle is called "sticking." By sticking to one's opponent, one harmonizes with his energy; one is safe from unexpected attack and is tuned in to his opponent's next move. It is this principle of harmonization/unconditional love that makes Tai Chi such an effective and unusual martial art form.

Phenoalynine works well as a combined agent with such chemicals as norepinephrine and adrenaline and dopamine. It works well being in the background and combining agent. Being very yin, it fools the body into thinking it's sugar, but is even more yin than sugar, and can upset the body's balance.

The sound of this scale is indeed sticky and too sweet, like ants on a fallen lollipop. The chromatic scale is always useful as a transition to other modes, as the half steps have not only an ambiguous quality but seem to want to lead somewhere (or follow somewhere).

The somewhere can be just about anywhere; it can blend easily with just about any other scale.

The power of Yin is as a bonding or combining agent. (Male bonding is an oxymoron, possible because men have feminine attributes, and vice-versa.)

Hexagram 3: Difficulty at the Beginning

C D Eb Fb G Ab Bb Cb

The image is of a blade of grass pushing against an obstacle as it pushes up out of the ground. "The hexagram indicates the way in which heaven and earth bring forth individual beings." Comparing the sound of this scale to that of a major scale, it is not difficult to perceive how the scale mirrors the meaning of the hexagram. The major scale leads effortlessly to the second tetra chord from the first because of the fourth note, F, which is led to from the third note, E, a half step. In this scale, Eb leads to Fb and leaves us with an awkward jump to the G that begins the second tetra chord. It gets much easier as we go along, however, and the Cb leads nicely back to the C. The hexagram reminds us that difficulties are part of life. If we expect them (remaining pessimistic about the nature of life), then we can remain optimistic about the nature of life.

Hexagram 4: Youthful folly

C Db Eb Fb   G Ab Bbb Cb

The Image is a spring at the foot of the mountains. However, instead of staying with a poetic feeling, we get youth and folly from the I Ching. The first part of the scale is rather somber, but the G-G#-A is almost comical.

Learning from the way in which water flows down, we find that this scale has a rather nice downward side to it. It's spiral nature.

Hexagram 5: Waiting (Nourishment)

I am reminded of *Siddartha* by Hesse. Siddhartha learned "how to fast and how to wait." In playing this scale, we notice that the scale seems to complete itself before returning to the root of the upper octave. It seems to resolve to B, the leading tone. Could that be a help in learning how to wait?

"Waiting is not mere empty hoping. It has the inner certainty of reaching the goal. Such certainty alone gives that light which leads to success..." "...Weakness and impatience can do nothing. Only a strong man can stand up to his fate, for his inner security enables him to endure to the end. This strength shows itself in uncompromising truthfulness. It is only when we have to the courage to face things exactly as they are, without any sort of self-deception or illusion, that a light will develop out of events, by which the path to success may be recognized.

Hexagram 6: Conflict

C Db Eb Fb / G A B C#

The trigrams for Heaven, pointing upward and the abysmal / water, leading downward compose this Hexagram.

Musically, it is the same; the first tetra chord is very commonly heard played in a downward direction, the upper some naturally leads up (to D). We have another conflict in that the tri-tone is between G and Db, wanting to resolve to an Ab or D root, neither of which exists in the scale. The I Ching has some good advice here for anyone in any situation involving conflict. You feel that you are in the right and are being obstructed.

"If a man is entangled in a conflict, his only salvation lies in being so clear-headed and inwardly strong that he is always ready to come to terms by meeting the opponent halfway. To carry on the conflict to the bitter end has evil effects even when one is in the right, because the enmity is then perpetuated."

As in the scale, resolution lies elsewhere.

Hexagram 7: The Army

C Db Eb Fb / G Ab Bbb Cbb

This represents the strength of water (danger) being held together with discipline on the outside.

Also, the strong line in the second place is of utmost importance—represents the general or leader of the army. This general is in the lower trigram, which is the *inner*, and thus, cannot be the absolute ruler of the trigram, which would be the fifth place. Therefore, it is a general, rather than commander in chief. Musically, we would say this scale is minor, but has major tendencies; and with the flat seventh, might be led to (or by) an element (F) not within the scale.

Hexagram 8: Holding Together

C Db Ebb Fbb / G Ab Bb Cb

This represents the way water flows together on the surface of the earth, always eventually joining all waters together. The

I-Ching speaks of a central figure, a center of influence; it goes on to state:

"If a man has recognized the necessity for union and does not feel strong enough to function as the center, it is his duty to become a member of some other organic fellowship."

The ear, being used to less constriction in the first half, would probably find its way to some other scale.

Hexagram 9: The Taming Power of the Small

C D E F# / G Ab Bb C

The commentary speaks of a restraining influence. The one weak line holds the strong lines in check, but it is not yet time for a change. This is a common political situation. Musically, the Ab seems to pull back. It literally pulls us back to G. The first tetra chord also leads to G; however, the Ab makes modulation to a G center too awkward.

Hexagram 10: Treading (on the Tiger's Tail)

C D E F / G A B C#

The weak and strong are in close proximity. I take this to mean two things: one is that if we are in a weak position, sometimes we have to just be brash enough to go ahead and step on the tail and take the consequences; the second is that if we are in a position of strength, we must behave with moderation and restraint.

Restraint in music is sometimes achieved by being economical with our materials—developing themes and figures completely before moving on or resolving completely. Can this scale, with its wandering/progressive tendency, help us to achieve this? We can created what is commonly referred to as a "tag ending" from chords built off this scale:

Dmin7 G7 emin7 A7

However, that seems like more of a substrata than a musical impulse to tread on any part of the tiger (musically); though, the more constrictive the form, the more likely one is to take chances, and the more likely the ear is to accept them.

12: C Db Eb Fbb   GABC

33: C Db Eb Fb   GABC

56: C Db Eb Fb   GABbC

Hexagram 12 Standstill, 33 Retreat, and 56 Travel carefully all refer to chemicals that stop or slow down functioning in the decoding process that occurs in the body, called "traffic codons."

One notices that they all have smaller intervals in the beginning and longer in the later part of the ascending scale. The small interval (the half-step) in certain situations is called a the leading tone. It leads into the next note. In general, smaller intervals create movement, seem to go somewhere; whereas the larger intervals are more static, amorphous and ambiguous. These particular scales seem to want to crawl back down to the bottom, rather than growing or ascending.

Hexagram 14: Possession in Great Measure

C D E F# G A Bb C

Lysine

The light of heaven that illuminates both good and evil. The weak line (through unselfish modesty) has the power to hold the strong lines.

Lysine prevents dwarfism, prevents effects of herpes and shingles. The scale, known as the Lydian Dominant, does indeed maintain its identity as a dominant sound by virtue of the half step (the flatted seventh). This scale is important because it is the closest to a "natural" scale formed by the overtones of the root.

Hexagram 28: Great Excess, Overbalancing Weight, Critical Balance

C Db Eb F G A B C

Aspartic Acid

The Hexagram represents a beam that is thick and heavy in the middle but weak at the ends. The situation is unstable.

Aspartic Acid eliminates a surplus of ammonia, improves stamina. Ammonia is produced by metabolism of protein. The ammonia is dealt with by the liver; therefore, an excess of protein can be hard on the liver.

It is easy to see the relationship of this scale to the Hexagram, especially if one thinks extremely literally. The chords of the II, III, V and VII are all *aumented chords*. The name augmented aside, the *sound* is heavy; by which I mean that it *feels* heavy. The reason for this is probably that the chord has a complicated nature: the major third creates peace and stability, and the augmented fifth creates the necessity for movement; the result is tension and complexity.

Hexagram # 30: Clinging, or Fire

CDEbF GABbC

Li means BRIGHTNESS or FIRE. The character of this scale is the two dark (broken) lines, which represent the darkness in the middle of the fire. Clinging is a description of the natural action of fire. (Fire's hunger is expressed by its clinginess).

The Dorian scale, containing the same notes (in the tempered system) as Bb major (BbCDEbFGA), is the "brightest" of the minor modes. (Play c minor—CDEbFGAbBbC—and listen for the difference). As for it being "fiery," listen to some (relatively) recent pieces written in the Dorian mode, such as John Coltrane's "Impressions" or Miles' "So What" or Freddie Hubbard's "Little Sunflower."

The character of the mode, besides the major sixth, is in the minor third and also the fact that it is symmetrical: the dominant is also a minor tetra chord. This gives the mode its "floaty" quality—not so "defined" as the minor. That is why it lends itself to "one chord" pieces. The I Ching says that that the character of the hexagram is determined by the dark lines. So it is the minor third which gives the mode its character. One might think that it is the major sixth. There is only one note difference between the Dorian mode and the Mixolydian (major/dominant) and only one note difference between the minor scale. Even though brighter than the minor, you can switch back and forth much less noticeably than between the Dorian and the Mixolydian.

Hexagram 32: Constancy, Continuity, Duration

CDbEbF GABbCb

Aspartic Acid

Union as an enduring condition; marriage as the coming together of eldest son and eldest daughter, the husband being the moving force outside, the wife inside being gentle (submissive).

The scale is not one of our "normal" modes built off of the diatonic scale. It sounds very plausibly like a gypsy scale and has a lot of character. It does hold together very well and should be a very useful scale.

Hexagram 35: Easy Progress

C Db Ebb Fbb   G A Bb C

Tryptophan

Ever-widening expansion. A man who is in a dependent position and whom others regard as an equal and are willing to follow. The image is of the sun rising and implies purification (from earthly things).

However Tryptophan works, we know it makes us sleepy. The scale has a hypnotic, lulling quality. Sleep, of course, is the great purifier and balancer. Note that the scale generally expands from smaller to wider intervals, and that the sound has a hypnotic effect.

Hexagram 38: Polarity, Opposition

C D E F G A Bb C (Mixolydian Mode)

Arginine

The Hexagram represents direct contrast—the lake which seeps downward and the flame which burns upward. Two women are living in the same house belonging to different men.

Arginine is given to men for energy and to combat impotence.

It is extremely interesting, as noted elsewhere, that this scale is the basis for the blues, especially the more primitive varieties, built almost entirely of dominant chords, which is built off this scale.

The scale contains the famous tritone or flatted fifth, denounced and forbidden by the early Church fathers (for obvious reasons).

Hexagram #41: Decrease, Sacrifice

C D E F G Ab Bbb Cb

The Hexagram refers to initial loss for latter gain. This is a start codon—begin a new task by cutting out unnecessary movement and waste. The energy saved will propel the new endeavor.

This, as opposed to the preceding scales, has the small intervals at the end. The last note is the leading tone to C, propelling toward a continuation.

Hexagram 58: Shared Joy

CDEF GABC (C major scale.)

Serine

"True joy rests on firmness and strength within, manifesting itself outwardly as yielding and gentle...When two lakes are joined they not dry up so readily, for one replenishes the other." The I-Ching points out that it is not the yielding, but the strong lines that give this hexagram its character. In terms of the structure of the scale, that would include the major third and major sixth and seventh.

The Hexagram correlates to the amino acid Serine, which helps the brain and nerves to function properly. Lack of this chemical causes unsteady nerves and poor functioning of the central nervous system. It has to do with connection between the brain and the central nervous system.

It is somewhat staggering to consider the amount of music written in the major mode.

It does indeed suggest brightness, joy, cheerfulness. Not all of this can be conditioned response to musical tradition: there has to be some objective truth to this joyfulness. One obvious reason is the fact that all of the notes but one are overtones of the root note.

This means that there is a minimal amount of tension in the scale. The tension that does exist—between the fourth and seventh notes (F and B), for example, can very easily and naturally be put to use within the myriad useable chord families produced by this scale.

Playing in the major mode, one can alternate between the tonic chord and the dominant chord. This is heard quite frequently in almost all kinds of music and perhaps is the reason for the way music in the major mode can retain interest, even within a two-chord context. This is very much like the two lakes replenishing each other—they are two tonal centers and it is very common for music of the European "classical" era to even modulate to the key of the dominant (GABCDEF#G) for a time, then return.

The major scale is also called a "diatonic" scale. This refers to the use of the sixth degree (A in the C scale) as an alternate tonal center. Perhaps this is the "other lake." It could possibly be argued that the F is the second lake. Both the F Major chord and the Aminor chord are used often as sources of variety and replenishment (note the blues form and the music of J.S. Bach). However, both of these chords, FAC and ACE are close enough to the C (CEG) that I do not believe that they give as much "replenishment" as GBD, or GBDF, which contains all of the tension notes of the C major scale. (Scale notes can be categorized in relation to a chord as either consonant ("resting") or dissonant ("moving" or tension.)

As far as the strong lines rather than the yielding giving the scale its character, this also is true in terms of the scale. The half steps merely express the pull toward the root and the fourth. The whole steps are what creates the major third in the tonic and dominant. This would be an apt description of the "character" of the scale.

Hexagram 41: Decrease, Sacrifice

C D E F   G Ab Bbb Cb

The Hexagram implies initial loss for later gain. The amino acid is what is called a start codon: a new task is begun by cutting out unnecessary movement and waste; the energy saved will propel the new endeavor.

The scale can be heard as a variation of the major scale. The compression of the second half increases the propulsion, in a very economical fashion, to the next note (C natural, the fundamental). However, on closer inspection, this compression, in which we have lost the top C, results in an A minor (Bbb minor) scale with a major 7th and a raised 6th—odd, but definitely workable, and the only way to get a minor scale on the 6th degree with a true dominant 5th chord (E7#13).

Hexagram 43: Breakthrough, Resoluteness

CDEF# GABC Lydian Mode

As result of resolute actions, conditions change and a breakthrough occurs. There is an implied danger here. The broken line at the top suggests the possibility of a single evil individual in a position of power.

The use of the Lydian scale in modern jazz definitely could be called a breakthrough The Lydian is the brightest of the scales, and is considered by some to be the "natural" major scale because the F# is contained tin the overtone series of C, whereas F is not. the Lydian scale can have an uplifting effect, in the sense of freedom from restraint, but the dangerous element can also be present. (Note the use of the Lydian scale in parts of Bernstein's score for "West Side Story.")

If we examine the row of fourths, we note that 7 of them make up a major scale. For instance, the C major scale is : BEADGCF. The song "Autumn Leaves" goes through a chord progression that touches all of those roots:

Bm7b5 E7 Am Dm7 G7 C F

Therefore, resolute action (resolving chords through the scale) leads to the fourth note in the scale, F, root of the Lydian scale.

Hexagram 49: Revolution

C D Eb F G A B C

Histidine

The image is of a lake with fire boiling up from underneath.

Too much of this substance found in brain of schizophrenics, yet too little will result in anger and tension. It has been used successfully to treat arthritis.

This scale is the melodic minor scale (in the upward direction). So, it leads to a higher vibrational quality. Whether this has any relevancy or not, the scale definitely has only an upward direction, like the fire beneath the water.

The hexagram originally referred to an animal's pelt, the molting and renewal with the seasons. Perhaps that refers to how Histidine works. Therefore, we have the higher vibrational quality making history into a spiral instead of a circle. The hexagram tells us how to deal with violent change or conflict in life—by being aware of the cyclical nature of all things.

In American popular music, this scale implies the dominant to the second degree of the scale, sometimes used in a "tag" or "tag ending," a chordal section usually at the end of a piece to dissapate the energy enough to end it, such as

/ cmin7 F7 dmin7 G7 / repeat / finally ending in Bb.

Hexagram 55: Full Abundance

C D Eb F   G A Bb Cb

(also) Histidine

The Hexagram expresses a peak that cannot last indefinitely

When this chord was heard

> ex: BDFBb   =G7+9

in Stravinsky's Rite of Spring, the year was 1913. This was the eve of the first World War and the Russian Revolution.

Hexagram 57. Penetrating—Wood / Wind

CDbEbF GAbBbC   (Phrygian mode)

"The penetrating quality of the wind depends on its ceaselessness." (See Hexagram 58, the interior Hexagram). Gentle persistence.

A doubled hexagram (see Dorian, Hexagram 30), it has a balanced, restful quality. The dominant (the chord built on the fifth step) is minor, and not the strong dominant that we experience in the major mode. This gives the scale its ambiguous, modal quality.

We in the Western world tend to think of "penetrating" as a violent act. Alternatively, we can think of the action of oil on wood, or gentle sunlight on the skin.

PART THREE: WHAT IT ALL MEANS

Chapter 9. General Principles

Everything is related

Everything is related to everything else (just about.)

The fundamental simplicity of the universe is incomprehensible except in terms of these seemingly complex relationships.

Vibration is the quality and action of internal motion—energy—creating time and space, which have no reality apart from vibration.

Because of the mathematical identity of music theory, the DNA permutations and the laws of human interaction as expressed in the I-Ching, the laws that apply to one field can apply to the others as well.

Such ideas as the Laws of Resonance, the Law of Octaves and the Law of Harmonics have wider applications than just music.

The Law of Resonance

A vibrating object produces a cyclic transference of energy through a medium. This is called sound, if we can hear it. Sound is independent of the object that created it. When this sound encounters another object in the medium or field, that object will vibrate at the same rate, depending on its physical properties. If the second object is tuned to the same pitch i.e., has the same structure/tension) as the first object, then it will vibrate longer.

The law of resonance is a true natural law; this is applicable to all situations, including human interactions. It may be that the law of attraction that we have heard so much about lately, is really a partial understanding of the law of resonance.

In nature, opposites attract. Like does not attract like; like, however, does resonate with like. Perhaps it amounts to the same thing; but just because someone loves filmmaking doesn't mean he or she will be invited to Sunday barbeque at the Spielberg's.

The Law of Resonance, however, is a valuable tool, especially when combined with understanding of her sisters, the Law of Octaves and the Law of Harmonics.

The Law of Harmonics

The Law of Harmonics is simple. When an object—any object, including a string from a violin or any other musical instrument—is set in vibratory motion, a certain pattern of large and small vibrations is created. This pattern is always the same, no matter the size or shape of the vibrating body.

Think of a dog shaking off after a bath: first the body—the large vibrations—then the tail—the small vibration, then the very tip of the tail—even smaller.

With a vibrating string, it happens all at once—the entire string vibrates, producing the fundamental tone and the resultant smaller vibrations, called harmonics, or overtones.

This can be demonstrated with a 15-20 foot rope, one end tied to a stationary object. Shaking the rope, first we get the fundamental, i.e., the entire rope vibrating as a whole.

(Imagine children playing jump rope—a time lapse picture of the rope itself.)

Then picture two jump rope images end to end—that is the string divided in half. (Picture a figure 8 on its side.)

Then, picture it in thirds, fourths, fifths, and so forth, theoretically to infinity, each smaller division producing a correspondingly higher pitch, which is in a very exact relationship to the fundamental. This is called the overtone series; and, though exactly the same overtone pitches or *harmonics* are produced by every fundamental of the same pitch, different harmonics will be emphasized according to the different structure of the vibrating body. Thus, we can tell the difference between the sound of a violin and a trumpet playing the same note. We can also tell the difference between the voice of our best friend on the phone and an automated sales call...usually.

Experiment with Piano

On a piano keyboard, push down the key that would be the e above middle c, but do not let it sound. This removes the damper from that note. Continue holding the key down and play the low c two octaves below middle c. The high "e" should be audible, since it is an overtone of the low C. Note that the piano is a tempered instrument, and the "e" that is the overtone of "C" is not exactly the same pitch as the high "e" on the instrument, even and especially if it is well tuned

It is difficult to separate the three laws of Resonance, Octaves and Harmonics, as they are so interrelated and interdependent. For instance, the overtones resonate with the fundamental, and vice versa. For example, if I play a high G, just a little squeak, the lower G will vibrate; and the lower G will easily set off the tiny overtone G.

This is because the higher G's are contained within the lower, as easily heard overtones. Though we can express the relationship graphically as a line or series of numbers, it is really more like the relationship of nesting dolls

The Law of Octaves

The non-musician will note that between any note called C and its octave—that is, the higher note that vibrates exactly twice as fast—are eleven other notes. An octave looks like this:

C C# D D# E F F# G G# A A# B C

The note C is distinguishable from all the other notes, but whether we double the vibrational rate, or double it twice or any number of times, the resultant tone will still be a C; an E still an E, and so forth.

Though the actual number of vibrations per second for any note is arbitrary and has changed slightly over the years, the doubling of any vibration will produce a higher version of the same note. This reflects the holographic or fractal nature of the universe. Philosophically, and in terms of human action, we say "as above, so below." We live our lives on many levels and dimensions; yet, in some ways, these levels and dimensions are the same and it would be inaccurate to judge one as being superior or inferior to another.

Yet, the Law of Octaves gives us a *directionality* to existence—an *orientation*, if you will; an orientation low to high, yet cyclical. I refer the reader to Volume Two of this series: Activation, the chapters on Tai Chi Chuan—orientation within the body, the root of the world, where the soul rises and sets.

Chapter 10. Snakes, DNA, Theology, Evolution and Prayer

Archetypes of the Body and Spirit

The relationship of dreams to mythology and religious imagery mirrors the relationship of the individual to the whole of humanity, if not to the whole of the Universe. Dreams, myths and exterior repositories of symbols such as religions all share certain symbols, such as the image or archetype of the snake.

The serpentine form of the DNA spiral suggests an explanation for the commonness of the snake in dreams and mythology as well. We may have noted how images appear in dreams that relate to the state of our bodies or our environment. For instance, a cold wind blowing open a window in the room might produce images of a wintry scene; fire might relate to the state of our liver or digestion.

Since all thought is necessarily a physical as well as mental process, might it be well to examine all areas of thought in light of these discoveries? Perhaps the structure of the DNA affects other areas of thought as well. Is it an accident that the structure of our music and a widely-used book of divination are based on the same internal structure as the DNA? As an organizational model or matrix, might we not find other uses for this pattern?

DNA and evolution

Crick, discoverer of DNA, indicates that it would be highly unlikely for the DNA to have been created spontaneously on earth. Life on this planet has been physically, chemically possible for only the past one billion years. According the Crick, the complexity level of even the simplest single-celled organism is too high to have developed in that period. The corollary to this thought is that the evolution of humanity is perhaps not as complex as a process as that to create a simple single cell.

The fact that every living organism on this planet shares the same DNA has led to some interesting speculation. Long before this discovery, a "primitive" South American myth tells of an intergalactic being hiding from a relentless enemy. It lands on

Earth and disguises itself as the variegated life-forms here.

Is it not true that we are more than what we can do, think or accomplish; and that which we can accomplish seems to come from a source other than ourselves, or at least a source apart or larger than our individual egos? We call this *inspiration.* What if our connection with others, with all life, extends deeper than we might be able to comprehend?

Cell Mutation Theory

Another theory of creation that is well out of the mainstream is Cell Mutation Theory. It postulates that all of our organs, cells and tissues were once individual beings that came together in cooperative harmony, or survival. I discuss this theory in greater detail in VOLUME TWO because this thought, if not necessarily having logical scientific provability, gives us a different way of looking at our bodies and how our bodies "think," which is not necessarily the way the "brain" thinks.

How would this fit in with the way the DNA works? The myriad forms joining into one organism seems like the exact opposite of the South American myth of one organism splitting into myriad forms. Theoretically, however, they both could have happened at a different times.

Convergent evolution—does it imply God?

Not only is the DNA the basic structure of the living cell—the same basic structure the same in all living things— but there is a convergence of specific features (such as the way eyes are formed) that make it appear that evolution is a planned process.

The question of god vs. evolution vs. alien transplants to my mind is not a question at all. We all want to know the unknowable, and isn't that what god is?

On the one hand, we have the "relgionists" pretending the Unknowable really isn't unknowable; on the other hand the "scientists" pretending the unknowable really isn't the Unknowable. In both cases, they are trying to put infinity in a box and chip away at it. It's just so big as to be overwhelming. But we all search in our own way, which is best; we are only truly off the path when we waste precious time judging the path of others or trying to block them.

The study of dreams and consciousness brings us quite naturally to the concept of the holographic field.

Chapter 11. The Holographic Field

Reality in 3-d

A holographic film produces an image in three dimensions. (For all we know, it may produce an image in more dimensions than three). Much can be learned about the nature of our reality through understanding the process of holography.

For instance, with two-dimensional film, if part of the film is missing, part of the image is missing. This is not true of the way the image is stored in holographic film. In the holographic process, if part of the in the film is cut off, that little piece will produce exactly the same exact image as the whole. This way of storing information is very similar to the way the brain stores and utilizes information—or the way we remember dreams. Missing part of the film will produce an image that will be less clear or less detailed, but the image will be there in totality.

The process of memory is similar—it is often easier to remember a name if we associate that person with another person of the same name. Note that we have added *more* information to be stored. However, by expanding the field, adding a new dimension, we have successfully increased connections with information that is already readily accessible to the brain.

Another example is how we remember dreams. Sometimes we do not remember until later, when something will trigger the memory. Again, we have widened the field to increase clarity.

In our study of the relationship of the I-Ching, music and the DNA, we have essentially created a field--a very wide one, indeed. The deeper we examine those three elements, the wider our field becomes and the clearer our picture of reality.

For All We Know...

Assuming that all we know of life and the universe is consciousness, that our tools for exploration—our senses and tool extensions—must be perceived on that "inner screen;" then why not see the entire universe as one conscious entity. The hologram makes a good model.

The recurring fractal images we see as the complexity of life unfolds approaches the infinite, approaches chaos. Think of the absolute beauty and mystery of a snowstorm—it is difficult to see the implicit order until we approach an individual snowflake. For those readers in tropical regions, each snowflake is unique, geometrically complex and symmetrically perfect.

Holographic Mechanics

Explaining how holograms are produced is beyond the scope of this book; however, it is worth mentioning the fact that besides the holographic film, one requires a coherent light source, otherwise known as a laser beam. This is a light source in which the photons march in organized rows as opposed to the scattered effect of ordinary light. This is a clear example of Yin and Yang, which will be discussed in more detail in Volume Two. The film is a receptive filed that contains the picture in encoded form—interference patterns—each little section of film containing the whole image, not just a part. This is the matrix—from the root *mater,* from which we get *material*, and *mother*. That is the Yin side of the equation.

On the Yang side, we have the coherent light source, which contains no information—it just *is*. This energy has long ago identified itself to us as Y*V*: "I AM THAT I AM."

Chapter 12. The Triangle

Were we to visualize a triangle, on one apex could be genetic code; on the other is the I-Ching; on the third angle is music.

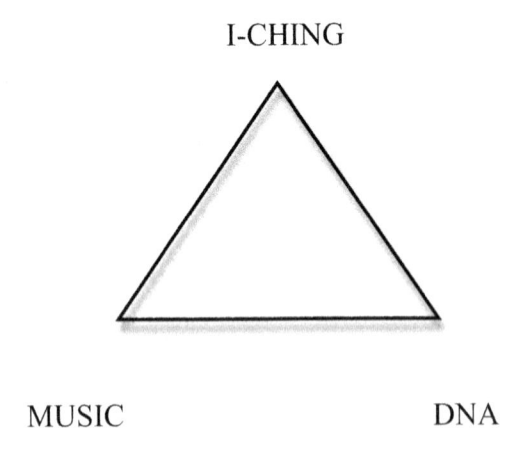

I-CHING

MUSIC   DNA

Apparently three areas of study--the I Ching, the genetic code and music—share a common language.

In the middle of the triangle lies perhaps Leonard Bernstein's "Unanswered Question"—what is beyond language? But first, we must ask, what is language?

Language is a tool for communication. What is the difference between communication and language? Communication is the process of information transfer. Language is the coding that makes possible the information/energy transfer. A punch or a kick is information/energy, as well as a kiss or e-mail. Therefore, the form of the message can have some objective importance. The nucleus of a cell can be communicated with by means of DNA. People respond to language and vibration as well as heat, color, light.

It is possible that people themselves or life itself is a form of energy/communication. Since most higher forms of language actually <u>store</u> energy/information, we could look at ourselves and all life as being a form of language.

Korzybski, in "Science and Sanity," which gives birth to the science of semantics, describes language as a process of abstraction.

Abstraction is the process of going from a generality to a specificity; or, vice versa. European languages start with the abstract. The word blue, for example, is abstract—merely a sound. The Chinese language, on the other hand, being pictographic rather than alphabetic, would start with picture symbols of several things that have the quality of blueness, and joins them together to express "blue." This is going from the concrete to the abstract. Neither is more adequate than the other, though the expatriate American poet Ezra Pound wrote a small, but intelligent treatise on why the Chinese language is an excellent medium for poetry; the reason being that it does go from the concrete to the abstract.

This discussion will be expanded upon in Volume Two, the meaning of the word Tai Chi, and Volume Three on the essence of poetry and art.

Chapter 13. Activation

The triangle is structurally the most stable of simple geometrical forms. However, by thinking of the triangle as a possible doorway, we can see the possibility of creating a progressive situation. This is the subject explored in our next volume: ACTIVATION.

The idea is very resonant with Chinese cosmology. The Wu Chu is the empty circle containing everything, infinite in all dimensions of time and space. It is represented by the empty circle; but on the human plane, it could be represented by this equilateral triangle. As soon as there is movement, however, Wu Chi become Tai Chi:

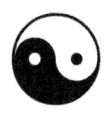

and the triangle becomes polarized as well. One angle is Yin, the other Yang, and the third angle the neutral controlling mechanism of Tai Chi itself.

Through this activation process, this doorway that we create *consciously*, we are able to transform our space into a space of healing and dynamic movement without losing the stability of the triangle.

This dynamism is implied *potentially* by the diagonal lines of the triangle; but through the efforts of many people and many lifetimes, humans have created a dynamic form to create and extend this activation. This is called Tai Chi Chuan—the Grand Ultimate Fighting Form. We can view it as a martial art, or a dance, or a poem, or a symphonic work, a tool for healing, or health; it is a tool for the activation of consciousness.

Though it is the principles underlying Tai Chi Chuan that will be our focus, we delve into the details of the form, as well as details on performance, lineage, and philosophy.

In truth, each movement of the Tai chi form is a key that unlocks a part of our genetic encodement, allows us to evolve to our fullest potential. Underlying this art form are principles that, when applied to other areas of life, have a liberating, enhancing effect. This is due to their universality, and due that, in the process of their unfolding, we do not approach consciousness directly.

We "train the mind to train the body." This is much the same as learning anything—how to dance, for instance, or draw, or play a musical instrument. The end result is that the mind is *already trained*. We do not have to think about it anymore, we "just do it." Is not this non-reflective, pure state of mind what we are seeking to begin with, as far as the mind is concerned. The fact that we can now do Tai Chi or play the bassoon, or have increased circulation is a by-product.

Without activation, any spiritual teaching, any philosophy is no better than a pile of paper with ink. Mohammed described the philosopher who did not live his philosophy as no better than a donkey carrying a load of books. The question, though, is *how?* We are told simply that it is not easy (a camel going through the eye of a needle). We are told to love our neighbor as ourselves, to turn the other cheek, to do unto others, etc. The skill required to do these things is not something we are born with or acquire easily, or learn at school or even the highest university. There have been too few Gandhis, too few Martin Luther King, Jrs. For most of us, successfully turning the other cheek, without succumbing to harm, requires that our learning be more than just ideas; it requires the transformation of individual consciousness that comes with the *activation* of those ideas. Meditation, training the mind, mental focus—these things are a life's work at the very least. A constant struggle?

This is why we may consider learning a martial art—to learn how *not* to fight. However, Kung-Fu—which means literally "hard work over a long period of time"—is not the only method of activation. We can also consider the principle of "pilgrimage." This is a journey to a place, a person or an idea—an alignment with principles or a tradition, or with a person.

A pilgrimage allows us direct contact with an energy or energies that somehow changes our perceptions, our focus; some would say it changes our DNA. It can take the form of a visit to a sacred space. There are places on the earth that are special; they have been pilgrimage spots for longer than recorded history. A pilgrimage can also take the form of meeting with a person; some feel going to see the Pope or a Tibetan lama at a live appearance has a great effect on the psyche—just being in that person's presence, something is transmitted. The same can be said for conventions of like-minded individuals. If, for example, we were to have a gathering of enough musicians, or chemists, or plumbers—because musicians and chemists and plumbers almost always learn from other musicians, chemists or plumbers—were we to trace the lineage of each individual back far enough, we would have in the room every master who ever lived.

Chapter 14. Completion

Universality

This concept of *pilgrimage* has a devotional aspect—the self merging into the large Ocean of Consciousness; as such, it connects with the idea of integration or COMPLETION, which is discussed in the final volume of "White Cloud Journey." Playing Tai Chi or engaging in any creative act that embraces and includes one's entire being—what we call *art*—COMPLETES the energy that created us. The circle that is completed is the circle of life itself.

Some ancient languages, the Tewa language for example, do not have a word for art; the activity was not separated from any other activity. We must assume that the lack of consciousness that made things not an art was not really part of their culture. If the word "beauty" is in the language, then we could make a verb out of that noun; but again, awareness of beauty implies allowing non-beauty into our lives and culture.

The existence of exceptional states—the so-called religious experience or "out-of-body" experience is common to all cultures. However, it is more accurate to call them "in-body experiences"—the body being the infinite realm that expresses the totality of what we are; at the very least, we should include the Earth as part of our body.

Art Forms

Art, whether we have a name for it or not, is the Journey's Return; because a journey in this sense is not just a journey *to* somewhere; it is incomplete without returning. In Islamic tradition, the word is *Ta'wil* (return); it is what makes a metaphor "work"; it is what makes a parable connect with life; it is the punch line to the joke.

Storytelling—the hero's journey, the nature and the principles of art—all of these can be integrated into our daily lives in such a way as to improve the experience for ourselves and others. Yet, there is more to it— there is a transcendent quality, also a mystery of where it possibly may come from.

We say that a work of art (or a religion or philosophy or a soft drink) is *universal*– meaning, it is useful or comfortable in many different situations, times and places, and for many different people and kinds of people. Another way of comprehending this is tuning in to the holographic nature of our world: taking a small bite off the corner of reality, we find it contains the flavor (informational nexus) of the whole universe.

Yet another way of perceiving this paradigm is *energetic*. We carry the energy of those forces that created us. Allowing those energies to resonate in our creations carries those same "creative" energies forward. The completion of the circle can take place within the individual or between two beings, within a group, or as energy transmitted by way of a work of art. This "thing that happens," this fleeting, momentary experience, is who and what we really are, not what we may seem to be.

The Impersonal Personal

The ancient martial art form of Tai Chi Chuan is a *personal* art form; more exactly, intra-personal; it is used to communicate within one's own personal universe of body/mind/spirit. Meditation in general is such an intra-personal art form. In the following volume of this work, we discuss these arts in more detail, as well as the *inter*-personal art forms of music, painting, cooking, etc. and the medical arts. Those latter forms connect people with one another. However, they have an intra-personal aspect as well; they create for the practitioner an inner life that in some cases transcends earthly limitations. Likewise, Kung-fu (martial arts) is both intra-personal and interpersonal. They first affect the self, but then extend the effect to others.

The Creative Imagination

The Creative Imagination is *first* a mode of perception. It is a way of perceiving truth. This truth is not an intellectual matter; it is determined by the *connection* of the mind/body/universe. If, for instance, we see the light in a person's eyes, or in our own, we can sense—not judge, but *know*—if that light is a true light. We can test its resonance with our totality. If cut off from that totality, then it is a distortion—worse than a lie, it creates the dance of evil. This dance is a solo dance—it only pretends to dance with others.

We cannot approach the development of the creative imagination directly. Rather, it is the part of learning we get from our teachers that comes from their lives: how their lives touch us and not from what they say or even do. Even that is only indirect, because the energy of the Creative Imagination comes *solely* from within the self.

We can only inspire others, not give them the fire of creation. The creative imagination is a form of self-activation; though unpredictable, its development is the subject of Volume Three of this book. The creative imagination is responsible for the return of the self *to* the self, the culmination of the White Cloud Journey.

Jeffrey Fisher

Known nationally and internationally as an award-winning composer, master musician, painter and lecturer, Jeffrey Fisher has been a writer since the age of nine, and started cooking at the age of five. He attended Pomona College as a Theatre/Eastern Philosophy student, and studied music and composition at SUNY at Buffalo and the Grove School, Studio City. Fisher's first exposure to Tai Chi Chuan was at NYU School of the Arts and later studied under Master Y.C. Chiang in Berkeley and Dr. Marshal Ho'o in California, as well as with many of Dr. Ho's students.

Fisher now lives on and maintains an off-the-grid retreat in the San Jacinto Mountains, practices Reflexology and Auricular Medicine, teaches Tai Chi Chuan, writes and plays the flute and bass violin. His four albums: Triumph of the Spirit, Fairy Tales – from the Ballet Hans Christian Andersen, Ocean of Consciousness, and Satyagraha – Songs of the Earth are all available on order from many of the large and small retailers; as are the following volumes of White Cloud Journey: Volume I: The Tao of Just About Everything, Volume II: ACTIVATION, Volume III: Completion.
www.HealingMusicoftheSouthwest.com, www.twobirdsflying.com.

THE TAO OF JUST ABOUT EVERYTHING

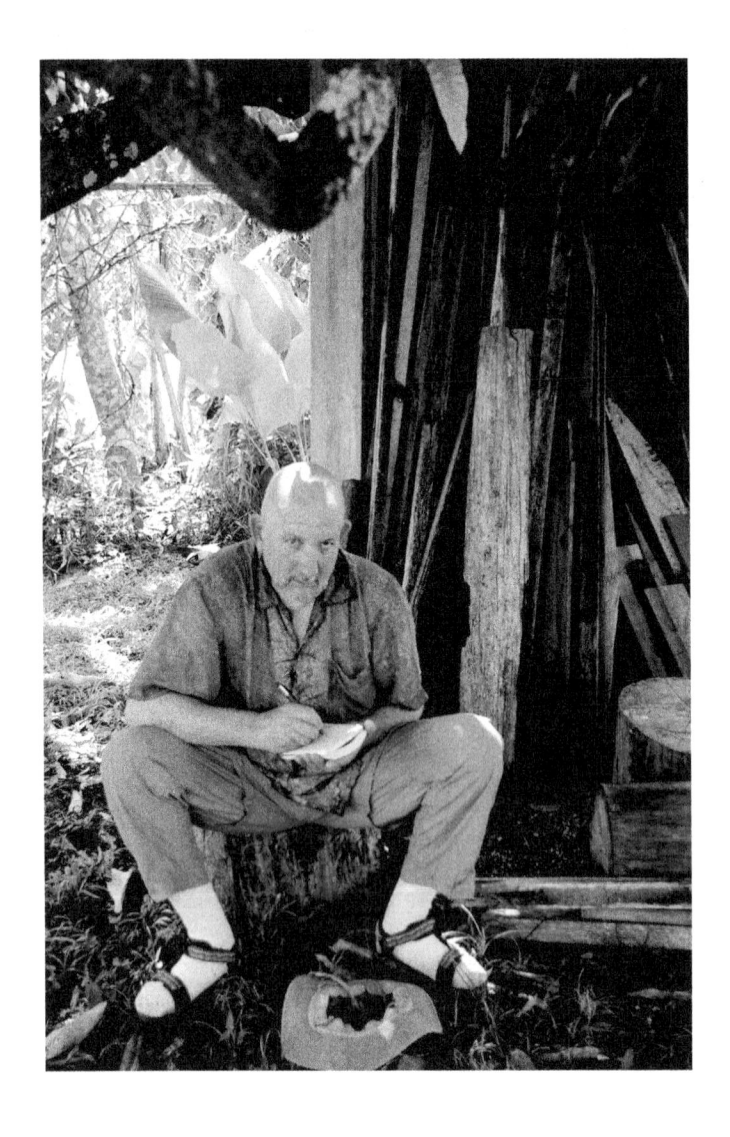

CPSIA information can be obtained at www.ICGtesting.com
Printed in the USA
BVOW08s0949060315

390595BV00012B/79/P